DECIPHERING DASH

A COMPREHENSIVE GUIDE TO DIETARY
APPROACHES TO STOP HYPERTENSION

A.D RAMS

Table of Contents

CHAPTER ONE

INTRODUCTION

The Dietary Approaches to Stop Hypertension (DASH) diet is a well-known dietary pattern that is suggested for improving general heart health and lowering high blood pressure, or hypertension. The DASH diet, created by the National Institutes of Health (NIH), places a focus on a balanced diet that is low in added sugars, saturated fats, and sodium and high in fruits, vegetables, whole grains, lean meats, and low-fat dairy products.

Numerous studies have shown how well the DASH diet works to decrease blood pressure and lower the risk of cardiovascular disease. It is a well-liked option for people trying to manage chronic health conditions and improve their diet since it places an emphasis on foods high in nutrients that are known to benefit heart health and general well-being.

We'll go over the fundamental ideas of the DASH diet, suggested food groupings, advantages for your health, and helpful hints for implementing it into your daily routine in this introduction. A flexible and evidence-based strategy to reaching your dietary objectives, the DASH diet can help you reduce blood pressure, strengthen your heart, or just change your eating habits.

A dietary plan called the DASH (Dietary Approaches to Stop Hypertension) diet was created to assist lower blood pressure and lessen the risk of heart disease, stroke, and hypertension. It places emphasis on restricting salt intake and eating a well-balanced variety of nutrient-rich meals. This is a summary of the DASH diet:

Fruits and Vegetables: Packed in fiber, vitamins, minerals, and antioxidants, fruits and vegetables are recommended as a part of the DASH diet. These meals assist in lowering blood pressure, strengthening the heart, and lowering the chance of developing chronic illnesses.

Whole Grains: An essential part of the DASH diet are whole grains such brown rice, quinoa, oats, and whole wheat bread. They offer fiber, minerals, vitamins, and phytonutrients that promote general health and heart health.

Lean Proteins: Fish, chicken, beans, lentils, tofu, and nuts are examples of lean protein sources that are part of the DASH diet. Compared to processed and red meats, these meals are lower in saturated fat and higher in protein, vitamins, minerals, and healthy fats.

Low-Fat Dairy: The DASH diet suggests low-fat dairy items such skim milk, yogurt, and cheese. They supply critical elements like protein, calcium, and others without the additional saturated fat that comes with full-fat dairy products.

Restricted Sodium: The DASH diet places a strong emphasis on cutting back on sodium because eating a diet heavy in sodium can raise blood pressure. Under the DASH diet, a maximum of 2,300 milligrams of salt should be consumed daily; for even further blood pressure reduction, 1,500 mg should be the ideal goal.

Moderate Consumption of Healthy Fats and Oils: The DASH diet promotes nuts, avocados, olive oil, and other foods high in healthy fats and oils in moderation. When ingested in moderation, these sources of monounsaturated and polyunsaturated fats support heart health.

Restrictions on Sweets and Added Sugars: The DASH diet calls for limiting sweets, sugar-filled drinks, and meals that include added sugar. These foods are high in empty calories and have been linked to blood sugar imbalances and weight gain.

Portion regulate: Although rigorous calorie counting is not necessary for the DASH diet, it is encouraged to assist regulate weight and calorie consumption. A healthy weight can be attained and maintained by eating thoughtfully and paying attention to portion amounts.

In general, the DASH diet encourages a varied and balanced pattern of eating that is low in processed foods, added sugars, saturated fats, and sodium and high in whole grains, fruits, vegetables, lean meats, and low-fat dairy. Adhering to the DASH diet has been shown to lower blood pressure, lower the risk of heart disease, and enhance general health and wellbeing.

Goals and intentions behind the DASH diet

The DASH (Dietary Approaches to Stop Hypertension) diet aims to lower blood pressure by making dietary modifications that also lessen the risk of hypertension, heart disease, and stroke. By encouraging a balanced eating pattern that prioritizes nutrient-rich foods while limiting sodium, saturated fats, and added sugars, the DASH diet seeks to accomplish these objectives.

The primary goals of the DASH diet are as follows:

Reduce Blood Pressure: Reducing blood pressure is the main goal of the DASH diet, especially for those who have hypertension or prehypertension. The DASH diet lowers systolic and diastolic blood pressure by emphasizing foods that are proven to lower blood pressure, such as fruits, vegetables, whole grains, lean meats, and low-fat dairy products.

Lower Risk of Hypertension: For people with normal or prehypertensive blood pressure, the DASH diet is intended to help avoid the development of hypertension. Those who maintain a well-balanced diet that is high in nutrients and low in sodium can eventually lower their chance of having high blood pressure.

Enhance Heart Health: Reducing the risk of cardiovascular disease and enhancing general heart health are two more goals of the DASH diet. The DASH diet lowers the risk of heart attack, stroke, and other cardiovascular problems by emphasizing heart-healthy foods like fruits, vegetables, whole grains, and lean proteins while restricting foods that worsen heart disease, like added sugars and saturated fats.

Encourage Overall Health and Well-Being: The DASH diet supports a balanced and diverse eating pattern in order to promote overall health and well-being, in addition to its targeted objectives regarding blood pressure and heart health. The DASH diet supports optimal health and lowers the risk of chronic diseases including diabetes, obesity, and some types of cancer by placing an emphasis on nutrient-rich foods that are high in vitamins, minerals, antioxidants, and fiber.

Promote Sustainable Lifestyle improvements: A key component of the DASH diet is encouraging long-term, sustainable lifestyle improvements. The DASH diet promotes people to build lifelong healthy habits by supporting a balanced eating pattern that is elastic and responsive to personal preferences and cultural customs.

The DASH diet aims to lower blood pressure, lessen the risk of heart disease and hypertension, improve general health and well-being, and support long-term lifestyle changes through dietary adjustments. The DASH diet's tenets can help people reach these objectives and enhance their quality of life.

Knowing About Hypertension and Its Effects

Elevated pressure in the arteries is a persistent medical disease called hypertension, or high blood pressure. Due to its high incidence and link to a higher risk of cardiovascular disease, stroke, kidney disease, and other consequences, it is a major global health concern. Effective prevention and management of hypertension require a thorough understanding of the condition's effects. This is a synopsis:

Blood Pressure Measurement: Systolic pressure, which is the upper number, and diastolic pressure, which is the lower number, are the two values that represent blood pressure in millimeters of mercury (mm Hg). Generally speaking, blood pressure less than 120/80 mm Hg is considered normal. When blood pressure continuously registers at 130/80 mm Hg or greater, hypertension is diagnosed.

Types of Hypertension: Two primary forms of hypertension are identified:

The most prevalent kind of hypertension, known as primary (essential) hypertension, appears gradually over time and has no clear cause. Numerous factors, including genetics, diet, lifestyle decisions, and environmental circumstances, frequently have an impact.

Secondary Hypertension: This kind of hypertension is brought on by a medicine or underlying medical condition. It might appear out of the blue and is frequently linked to illnesses like kidney disease, hormone imbalances, or specific drugs.

Risk variables: A number of variables raise the possibility of hypertension, such as:

Age: As people age, their risk increases, and older folks are more likely to have hypertension.

Family History: Those who have a history of hypertension in their families are more vulnerable.

Lifestyle Factors: Poor eating, inactivity, binge drinking, and smoking are among the unhealthy lifestyle choices that lead to high blood pressure.

Obesity: Having a high body mass index or being fat raises the risk of hypertension.

Chronic Conditions: Hypertension risk can be raised by chronic conditions such renal disease, diabetes, and sleep apnea.

Impact on Health: If untreated, hypertension can have major negative effects on one's health. It strains the arteries, heart, and other organs, raising the possibility of:

Cardiovascular Disease: One of the main risk factors for heart attacks, strokes, and heart disease is hypertension.

Chronic renal disease or kidney failure can result from high blood pressure's long-term harm to the kidneys.

Damage to the Eyes: High blood pressure can harm the blood vessels in the eyes, resulting in impaired vision or even blindness.

Cognitive Decline: In older persons, dementia and cognitive decline are more likely to occur when chronic hypertension is present.

Prevention and Management: The best ways to avoid and control hypertension are through lifestyle changes. Among them are:

Adhering to a nutritious diet, like the DASH (Dietary Approaches to Stop Hypertension) diet, which places a focus on whole grains, fruits, vegetables, lean meats, low-fat dairy, and minimal amounts of salt, saturated fats, and added sweets.

taking part in regular exercise.

keeping a healthy weight in mind.

reducing the amount of alcohol consumed.

Giving up smoking.

Using stress-reduction and relaxation methods to manage stress.

taking prescription drugs as instructed by a medical practitioner, if required.

A prevalent and dangerous medical disorder having major effects on one's health is hypertension. It is vital to comprehend the risk factors, health effects, and preventive and management techniques associated with cardiovascular disease in order to enhance heart health and lessen its burden. The mainstays of hypertension treatment and prevention include effective medication therapy, lifestyle changes, and routine blood pressure monitoring.

Fundamental Ideas of the DASH Diet

Based on a number of fundamental ideas, the DASH (Dietary Approaches to Stop Hypertension) diet aims to reduce blood pressure and enhance general health. These guidelines have a focus on eating meals high in nutrients and reducing your intake of added sugars, saturated fats, and sodium. The following are the main ideas behind the DASH diet:

Place an Emphasis on Fruits and Vegetables: The DASH diet promotes fruit and vegetable consumption as the cornerstone of a balanced diet. Rich in vitamins, minerals, antioxidants, and fiber, these foods support general health by lowering blood pressure and lowering the risk of heart disease. Make it a daily goal to eat a range of vibrant fruits and veggies.

Select Whole Grains: A keystone of the DASH diet is whole grains. They offer fiber, minerals, vitamins, and phytonutrients that promote general health and heart health. Select whole grain products over refined grains, such as brown rice, quinoa, oats, whole wheat bread, and whole grain pasta.

Incorporate Lean Proteins: A key component of the DASH diet is lean protein sources. Choose lean protein sources instead of red meat and processed meats, like fish, chicken, beans, lentils, tofu, and nuts. These foods are lower in saturated fat. These meals supply vital nutrients like zinc, iron, and protein without the extra cholesterol and saturated fat.

Limit Sodium Intake: One of the main goals of the DASH diet is to help lower blood pressure by limiting sodium intake. Excessive consumption of salt can raise the risk of heart disease and contribute to hypertension. Try to keep your daily sodium consumption to 2,300 mg, ideally aiming for 1,500 mg to further lower your blood pressure. Steer clear of adding extra salt to your meals and go for low-sodium or no-salt choices instead.

Minimize Saturated Fats and Added Sugars: The DASH diet advises avoiding saturated fats and added sugars since they raise the risk of heart disease and other health issues. Select low-fat dairy products, lean protein sources, and healthy fats like nuts, avocados, and olive oil. Eat less sweets, sugar-filled drinks, and foods with added sugar.

Practice Portion Control: To prevent overindulging and control calorie intake, pay attention to serving and portion sizes. When portioning out foods, especially high-calorie goods like nuts, oils, and starchy carbohydrates, use measuring cups, spoons, and food scales as needed. Throughout the day, eating smaller, more frequent meals can also aid in regulating appetite and avert overindulgence.

Keep Yourself Hydrated: To maintain general health and stay hydrated, sip lots of water throughout the day. Water facilitates normal bodily system functioning, aids in digestion, and helps control appetite. Try to drink eight to ten glasses of water a day, or more if it's hot outside or you're physically active.

People can enhance their general health and well-being, lower their blood pressure, and lessen their risk of heart disease by adhering to these fundamental DASH diet guidelines. The DASH diet limits added sugars, saturated fats, and sodium while promoting a nutrient-dense, well-balanced, and diverse eating pattern. It's a sustainable and adaptable method of eating healthily that can help people of various ages and circumstances.

Food Groups and Servings for the DASH Diet

Dietary Approaches to Stop Hypertension, or DASH, diet places a strong emphasis on a balanced diet that consists of a range of foods high in nutrients from several food groups. The purpose of these dietary groups and suggested serving sizes is to assist people in reducing blood pressure and enhancing their general health. The following lists the food groups and suggested serving sizes for the DASH diet:

Fruits: Because of their high vitamin, mineral, antioxidant, and fiber content, fruits are an essential part of the DASH diet. Make it a daily goal to eat a range of fruits. Suggested portions:

Four to five portions daily

One medium apple, one medium banana, half a cup of berries, or three-quarters of a cup of 100% fruit juice are examples of one serving.

Vegetables: Low in calories and high in fiber and other nutrients, vegetables are another important part of the DASH diet. Make it a daily goal to eat a range of vibrant vegetables. Suggested portions:

CHAPTER TWO

1/2 cup cooked veggies, 1 cup raw leafy greens, or 3/4 cup vegetable juice are some examples of one serving.

Grains: Due to their high fiber content and nutritional advantages, whole grains are advised on the DASH diet. Whenever feasible, opt for whole grains rather than refined ones. Suggested portions:

6–8 portions daily

One ounce of whole grain cereal, half a cup of cooked brown rice or quinoa, or one slice of whole wheat bread are some examples of one serving.

Lean Proteins: Rich in critical nutrients without the added saturated fat of fatty meats, lean protein sources are a crucial component of the DASH diet. Select protein sources that are low in fat, such as fish, chicken, beans, lentils, tofu, and nuts. Suggested portions:

two or fewer portions of fish, poultry, or meat each day

two to three servings of legumes, seeds, or nuts each week

Three ounces of cooked meat, poultry, or fish—roughly the size of a deck of cards—is an example of one serving of any of these foods.

Low-Fat Dairy: Unlike full-fat dairy products, which include an excess of saturated fat, low-fat dairy products contain calcium, protein, and other necessary elements. Pick selections that are fat-free or low-fat. Suggested portions:

two to three portions daily

One cup of skim or 1% milk, one cup of yogurt, or 1.5 ounces (about the size of four dice) of cheese are examples of one serving.

Fats & Oils: Although they should be avoided in moderation when following the DASH diet, trace amounts of healthful fats can be consumed. Opt for healthy fats like those found in almonds, avocados, and olive oil. Suggested portions:

two to three portions daily

One-eighth of an avocado, one teaspoon of olive oil, or one tablespoon of nuts or seeds are a few examples of one serving.

Sweets and Added Sugars: Because they are rich in calories and low in nutrients, sweets and added sugars should be consumed in moderation when following the DASH diet. Desserts, sugar-filled drinks, and added-sugar foods should be avoided. Suggested portions:

Five portions or fewer every week

One little cookie, one tablespoon of sugar, or half a cup of ice cream are some examples of one serving.

On the DASH diet, people can attain a healthy and well-balanced eating pattern that promotes general health and lowers blood pressure by adhering to these suggested servings from each food group. Depending on dietary restrictions, tastes, and individual calorie requirements, serving quantities may need to be adjusted.

Advantages of the DASH Diet for Health

There are several health advantages to the DASH (Dietary Approaches to Stop Hypertension) diet, especially when it comes to heart health and the avoidance of chronic illnesses. The DASH diet has the following main health advantages:

Reduces Blood Pressure: Reducing blood pressure is one of the main objectives of the DASH diet, especially for those who have hypertension or prehypertension. Studies have repeatedly demonstrated that even in as short as two weeks, adherence to the DASH diet can result in notable drops in both systolic and diastolic blood pressure. The DASH diet minimizes sodium consumption and places an emphasis on nutrient-rich foods to assist maintain healthy blood pressure levels.

Lowers chance of Hypertension: The DASH diet is useful in lowering blood pressure in people with normal or prehypertensive blood pressure, as well as in lowering their chance of developing hypertension. By preventing high blood pressure from developing over time, the DASH diet can minimize the need for medication and lessen the risk of heart disease and stroke.

Enhances Heart Health: A number of heart health indicators, such as inflammation, triglycerides, and cholesterol levels, have been linked to benefits while following the DASH diet. The DASH diet lowers the risk of heart disease and other cardiovascular problems by prioritizing heart-healthy foods such fruits, vegetables, whole grains, lean proteins, and healthy fats while reducing sodium, saturated fats, and added sweets.

Supports Weight Management: A healthy weight can be reached and maintained by following the DASH diet, which is beneficial for weight management. The DASH diet encourages a balanced eating pattern that is high in foods high in nutrients and low in foods high in calories.

This helps to regulate appetite, lessen cravings, and support long-term, sustainable weight loss.

Enhances Insulin Sensitivity: Adhering to the DASH diet may enhance insulin sensitivity while lowering the chance of type 2 diabetes. The DASH diet lowers added sugars and refined carbs and increases whole grains, fruits, vegetables, and lean proteins. This helps to improve metabolic health and regulate blood sugar levels.

Enhances General Health and Well-Being: In addition to lowering blood pressure, the DASH diet is linked to a host of additional health advantages, such as better immune system performance, decreased inflammation, and improved digestive health. The DASH diet promotes general health and lowers the risk of chronic diseases including cancer, osteoporosis, and neurological disorders by offering vital nutrients, antioxidants, and fiber.

All things considered, the DASH diet is a comprehensive, scientifically supported way of eating that has many positive health effects. People can enhance their general health, reduce their risk of chronic diseases, and live longer by adhering to the DASH diet's guidelines and selecting nutritious foods.

Getting the DASH Diet Started

Starting the DASH (Dietary Approaches to Stop Hypertension) diet is an easy and efficient strategy to reduce blood pressure and enhance general health. The following actions will assist you in beginning the DASH diet:

Educate Yourself: Learn about the DASH diet's tenets, which include minimizing salt, saturated fats, and added sugars and placing a focus on fruits, vegetables, whole grains, lean meats, and low-fat dairy products. Making informed meal decisions will be made easier if you are aware of the main elements of the DASH diet.

Evaluate Your Present Diet: Examine your present eating patterns and note any areas in which you might improve. For a few days, keep a meal journal to monitor your consumption and assess how much added sugar, sodium, and saturated fat you're consuming. This will assist you in determining what needs to be changed.

Establish Achievable Goals: Make sure your diet includes foods that are DASH-friendly by setting attainable goals. Begin by implementing minor adjustments, like increasing the amount of veggies you eat or selecting nutritious grains over refined ones. Over time, progressively boost the amount of DASH-friendly meals you eat.

Load Up on DASH-Friendly meals: Stock your kitchen with healthy grains, fruits, veggies, lean meats, low-fat dairy products, and other DASH-friendly meals. Whenever feasible, go for whole, fresh foods rather than processed or packaged ones, which are sometimes heavy in added sugars and sodium.

Plan Your Meals: Make sure you have DASH-friendly options on hand by scheduling your meals and snacks ahead of time. Incorporate a range of foods from every food group and strive for meals that are balanced and offer a variety of nutrients. Plan your menu using DASH-friendly recipes and meal ideas as a guide.

Practice Portion Control: To prevent overindulging and control calorie intake, pay attention to serving and portion sizes. When portioning out foods, especially high-calorie goods like nuts, oils, and starchy carbohydrates, use measuring cups, spoons, and food scales as needed.

Lower Sodium Intake: Opt for lower-sodium foods and season food using herbs, spices, and other seasonings rather than salt to gradually cut down on your sodium intake. Fresh, whole foods are preferable whenever feasible; processed and packaged foods, which are frequently heavy in sodium, should be used sparingly.

Keep Yourself Hydrated: To maintain general health and stay hydrated, sip lots of water throughout the day. Water facilitates normal bodily system functioning, aids in digestion, and helps control appetite. Try to drink eight to ten glasses of water a day, or more if it's hot outside or you're physically active.

Seek Support: To keep yourself accountable and motivated while following the DASH diet, enlist the aid of friends, family, or support groups. Inform people about your objectives and solicit their assistance in choosing well.

Track Your Progress: Regularly check your weight, blood pressure, and other health indicators to stay informed about your progress. Enjoy your victories and practice self-compassion while you progress through the DASH diet. Keep in mind that over time, little adjustments can have a large impact.

You may lower your blood pressure, lessen your risk of chronic diseases, and improve your general health by implementing these simple measures and adding DASH-friendly items to your diet. With the DASH diet, start small, maintain consistency, and reap the rewards of a healthy way of living.

Planning Meals and Using Sample Menus

A key component of successfully implementing the DASH (Dietary Approaches to Stop Hypertension) diet is meal planning. You can make sure you're eating a range of nutrient-dense foods and staying under suggested limits for sodium, saturated fat, and added sugar by organizing your meals in advance. Here are some sample menus and instructions for making a DASH-friendly meal plan to get you started:

Tips for Meal Planning:

Eat a Range of Foods: Try to incorporate items from every dietary group into your meals, such as whole grains, fruits, vegetables, lean meats, low-fat dairy, and whole grains.

Try to arrange your plate such that fruits and veggies make up half of it, whole grains make up quarter, and lean protein sources make up the other quarter. This will assist you in preparing wholesome, well-balanced meals.

Select Whole Foods: Steer clear of processed and packaged foods, which are frequently heavy in sodium, saturated fats, and added sugars, and instead choose for fresh, whole foods wherever available.

Cook at Home: Preparing meals in your own kitchen gives you more control over the ingredients and serving amounts, which makes sticking to the DASH diet simpler.

Make a grocery list to make sure you have everything you need on hand before you go grocery shopping. This will help you plan your meals and snacks.

Watch Your Portions: To prevent overindulging and control calorie consumption, be mindful of serving and portion sizes.

Examples of Menus

First Day:

Breakfast consists of whole grain toast with avocado slices and Greek yogurt covered with a mixture of berries and honey.

Hummus-topped carrot sticks for a snack.

Lunch is a salad of grilled chicken, mixed greens, cucumbers, cherry tomatoes, and balsamic vinaigrette.

Snack: Almond butter on sliced apples.

Steamed broccoli, quinoa pilaf, and baked fish with lemon and dill for dinner.

Day 2:

Breakfast consists of heated oatmeal with skim milk, chopped walnuts, and sliced banana on top.

Snack: strawberries cut into slices with Greek yogurt.

Lunch consists of a whole wheat tortilla rolled with avocado, turkey, tomato, and mustard.

Snack: Peanut butter-covered celery sticks.

Supper is brown rice topped with stir-fried tofu and mixed veggies.

Day Three:

Breakfast consists of whole grain pancakes with a dollop of Greek yogurt and fresh berries on top.

Snack: Pineapple pieces mixed with cottage cheese.

Lunch consists of a quinoa salad dressed with lime vinaigrette, black beans, corn, chopped bell peppers, and cherry tomatoes.

A handful of almonds as a snack.

Dinner is steamed asparagus, whole wheat couscous, and grilled shrimp skewers with bell peppers and onions.

You are welcome to combine or subtract meals from this list to make a custom DASH-friendly menu that suits your needs. To fully benefit from the DASH diet, remember to consume enough of fruits, vegetables, whole grains, lean proteins, and low-fat dairy products while reducing your intake of salt, saturated fats, and added sweets.

Advice for Social Events and Eating Out

It can be difficult to stick to a DASH (Dietary Approaches to Stop Hypertension) diet when dining out or at social events, but it is totally doable with some preparation and awareness.

CHAPTER THREE

The following advice will help you maintain your DASH diet while navigating social events and eating out:

Eating Outside:

Investigate Restaurants: Check internet menus to determine if a restaurant has DASH-friendly selections before making a decision. These days, a lot of restaurants have nutritional information on their websites to assist you in making decisions.

Make A Wise Choice: Select eateries that provide a range of healthful selections, including salads, baked or grilled proteins, and vegetable-based meals. Instead of frying or overly sauced food, opt for items that are baked, grilled, or steamed.

Request Modifications: Don't be hesitant to request that menu items be changed to make them more DASH-friendly. Ask for items to be served with fewer sauces on the side, less oil, and less salt. The majority of eateries are happy to fulfill specific requests.

Be Aware of Portion Sizes: Generally speaking, restaurant servings are larger than those you might find at home. To aid with portion control, think about splitting an entree with a dining partner or asking for a half serving.

Be Aware of Side Dishes: Recognize that side dishes and accompaniments can add a substantial amount of calories and sodium to your diet. Steamed veggies, side salads with vinaigrette dressing, and brown rice are healthier alternatives to fries or mashed potatoes.

Limit Alcohol: Beverages with added sugars and high calorie content should be avoided. Reduce your alcohol use and go for lighter options like wine, light beer, or soda water or diet soda mixed cocktails.

Social Events:

Bring a dish: Offer to bring a meal that is DASH-friendly to share if you're going to a potluck or other function. This lets people sample the delectable tastes of the DASH diet and guarantees that you'll always have at least one healthy option available.

Eat Beforehand: If you think there might not be as many healthy options during a social gathering, think about having a filling breakfast or snack first. This can lessen the likelihood of overindulging or making poor decisions due to hunger.

Moderation is key when it comes to high-calorie or high-sodium foods, even though it's acceptable to indulge occasionally. Don't overindulge in your favorite sweets; instead, enjoy tiny servings.

Keep Hydrated: To stay hydrated and help regulate hunger, drink lots of water during social gatherings. Sometimes people confuse their thirst for hunger, which results in needless munching.

Prioritize Socialization: Prioritize spending time with friends and family during social gatherings rather than making food the center of attention. Play games, take walks, or partake in other common hobbies as alternatives to eating-related activities or talks.

You can enjoy eating out and social gatherings without sacrificing your DASH diet objectives if you heed these recommendations. Always keep in mind that moderation and consistency are essential, and don't be too hard on yourself if you occasionally choose less healthful selections.

Prioritizing your health and well-being while still indulging in life's joys is crucial.

Integrating Physical Activity and Exercise

A healthy lifestyle should include frequent exercise and physical activity in addition to following the DASH (nutritional Approaches to Stop Hypertension) diet's nutritional guidelines. Exercise is important for controlling blood pressure, lowering the risk of heart disease, and enhancing general health and wellbeing in addition to helping with weight management. The following advice can help you maintain a DASH diet while adding exercise and physical activity to your daily routine:

Choose Physical Activities You Enjoy: Make a list of the things you enjoy doing physically. Find enjoyable and satisfying activities to engage in, such as walking, swimming, bicycling, dancing, or sports.

Establish Achievable and Realistic Goals: Whether your aim is to walk for thirty minutes a day, go to a fitness class three times a week, or walk a specific number of steps every day, make sure it is realistic. As your fitness level increases, progressively raise your initial, manageable goals.

Make It a Habit: Plan your physical activity and workout sessions into your weekly or daily schedule, the same way you would any other appointment or obligation. To see results and benefit from exercise's health benefits, consistency is essential.

Mix It Up: To keep things fresh and avoid monotony, mix up your routine by including other activities. To work different muscle groups and keep your body challenged, try a variety of exercise routines, such as aerobic, strength training, flexibility exercises, and balancing exercises.

Keep Moving Throughout the Day: Even when you're not doing formal exercise, try to find ways to get in some movement throughout your day. Instead of using the elevator, use the stairs, park further away from your destination, clean the house, or take short walks throughout the day.

Listen to Your Body: During exercise, pay attention to how your body feels and modify the intensity or length of your workout as necessary. As your fitness increases, it's acceptable to start out slowly and progressively increase the duration and intensity of your workouts.

Keep Hydrated: To stay hydrated and promote peak performance, drink lots of water prior to, during, and after exercise. Exercise performance can be hampered by dehydration, and heat-related illnesses are more likely to occur.

Warm Up and Cool Down: To ensure that your muscles and joints are ready for activity, warm up properly before beginning any workout. Then, at the end of your session, cool down to aid in your body's recovery. Stretching can increase range of motion and lower the chance of injury.

Have Reasonable Expectations: Be kind to yourself and don't count on seeing results right away. Strength, endurance, and fitness are things that require time and practice. Honor your accomplishments along the road and concentrate on the beneficial adjustments you're making for your well-being.

Seek Support: To increase motivation and accountability, think about working out with a buddy, relative, or personal trainer. Exercise can be more fun when you workout with a partner, and it can also help you stick to your fitness objectives.

You may maximize the health benefits of the DASH diet and boost your general health and well-being by including regular exercise and physical activity in your regimen. To make exercise a sustainable and pleasurable part of your lifestyle, keep in mind to start out cautiously, set realistic goals, and engage in fun activities.

Tracking Development and Making Modifications

Achieving success with the DASH (Dietary Approaches to Stop Hypertension) diet and any lifestyle modifications you're undertaking requires tracking your progress and making necessary adjustments. Here's how to keep an eye on your development and make the required corrections:

Tracking Development:

Check Your Blood Pressure Frequently: If you're managing your hypertension with the DASH diet, make sure to check your blood pressure frequently at home or during appointments with your doctor. To monitor your development over time, keep a record of your readings.

Monitor Your Food Intake: Maintain a food journal to record your daily intake of food and liquids. You may use this to spot trends, keep an eye on how much sodium you consume, and make sure you're adhering to the DASH diet recommendations.

Monitor Your Weight: Pay attention to your weight on a regular basis, but keep in mind that changes might not show up right away. If necessary, strive for lasting weight loss and acknowledge your little accomplishments along the road.

Evaluate Your Energy Levels: Keep a note of your feelings during the day. Better general health, elevated energy levels, and happier moods can all be indicators that your dietary and lifestyle modifications are working.

Examine Other Health Markers: Keep an eye on blood pressure, weight, cholesterol, blood sugar, and physical fitness in addition to these two primary health indicators. These indicators can provide important information about your general well-being and development.

Making Modifications:

Regularly Evaluate Your Progress: Give yourself some time to see if you're accomplishing your objectives by reviewing your progress. Think back on what's going well and any areas that might require modification.

Determine Potential Improvement Areas: If the outcomes you were hoping for aren't materializing, determine what may be done better. Are you adhering to the DASH diet recommendations consistently? Exist any particular foods or routines that might be impeding your progress?

Modify Your Diet as Necessary: If you're not getting the expected outcomes, think about modifying your diet to more closely follow the DASH guidelines. While reducing your consumption of sodium, saturated fats, and added sugars, concentrate on consuming more fruits, vegetables, whole grains, lean proteins, and low-fat dairy products.

Change Your Workout Routine: If you're not reaching your fitness objectives, you might want to think about changing your workout regimen. To keep things fresh, experiment with varying the duration, intensity, or frequency of your workouts. You may also try adding new exercises.

Seek Support: Don't be afraid to ask a qualified nutritionist, fitness trainer, or healthcare expert for assistance if you're finding it difficult to go forward on your own. They can offer you individualized advice and assistance to help you accomplish your objectives.

Be Patient and Persistent: Recall that it takes time and consistency for lifestyle modifications to produce desired effects. Even if you're not making improvements right away, practice self-compassion and persistence. Keep your attention on your long-term health and well-being while acknowledging your accomplishments along the road.

You can stick to your DASH diet objectives and manage your health and well-being in the long run by keeping a close eye on your progress and making any adjustments. Remain dedicated to implementing healthy habits that will support your health, keeping in mind that little adjustments can add up to significant outcomes over time.

Testimonials and Success Stories

Success stories and endorsements can serve as a source of inspiration and encouragement for anyone contemplating or presently adhering to the DASH (Dietary Approaches to Stop Hypertension) diet. Here are some illustrations of DASH diet success stories and testimonies from people who have benefited from it:

John's Path to Lower Blood Pressure: For years, John battled hypertension and needed medicine to control his blood pressure. Following the DASH diet and implementing lifestyle modifications, such as consistent exercise and stress reduction practices, John achieved notable reductions in his blood pressure and decreased dependency on medication. He has shed some pounds, gained energy, and his general health has improved.

Sara's Story of Success: Throughout her adult life, Sara battled with her weight, putting her at risk for heart disease and other health issues. Sara decided to adhere to the DASH diet's recommendations and make regular exercise a part of her routine after learning about its advantages. She eventually reduced her blood pressure, raised her cholesterol, and shed more than 50 pounds. Sara is motivated to sustain a long-term healthy lifestyle by her DASH diet success.

Tom's Transformation: Initially dubious about the DASH diet, Tom made the decision to give it a shot after running into health problems associated with his elevated blood pressure. Tom modified his diet gradually under the supervision of a trained nutritionist, emphasizing the consumption of whole grains, fruits, and vegetables at the expense of sodium. He also began to include regular exercise in his daily regimen. Tom's blood pressure and general health significantly improved in a matter of months. He now advises everyone wishing to strengthen their heart health to follow the DASH diet.

Emily's Path to Better Health: For years, Emily battled yo-yo dieting and unhealthy eating practices, which resulted in weight gain and health problems. Emily made the decision to try the DASH diet after hearing about it from a friend. She loved the range of foods allowed by the DASH diet and found it to be an easy diet to follow. Emily made long-lasting lifestyle adjustments and adhered to the DASH principles with the help of her friends and family. Since then, she has reduced her weight, raised her blood pressure, and felt happier and more energized than before.

These endorsements and success stories demonstrate the beneficial effects that the DASH diet may have on people's health and general wellbeing. Many people's blood pressure, weight, and general health have significantly improved by adopting the DASH principles and changing their lifestyle. These tales serve as a reminder that long-term success with the DASH diet is achievable with perseverance, support, and dedication.

Summary

In summary, the DASH (Dietary Approaches to Stop Hypertension) diet is a sustainable lifestyle strategy that supports general health and well-being, not just a short-term eating plan. The DASH diet offers many health benefits, such as lower blood pressure, a lower risk of heart disease, weight management, and improved overall health. It does this by emphasizing nutrient-rich foods like fruits, vegetables, whole grains, lean proteins, and low-fat dairy products while limiting sodium, saturated fats, and added sugars.

We've covered a lot of ground in this tutorial on the DASH diet, including its foundational ideas, advantages for health, advice on meal planning, sample menus, and methods for combining exercise and eating out. We've also heard uplifting success stories and testimonies from people who have followed the DASH diet and seen improvements in their lifestyle and health.

When you start your personal DASH diet journey, keep in mind that tiny changes over time can have a big impact. Progress takes time. Remain dedicated to making healthful decisions, pay attention to your body, and ask for help when you need it. You can attain long-term success with the DASH diet and lead a happier, healthier life if you are committed to it, follow it consistently, and have an optimistic outlook.

THE END